Perfect Vision Diet

The Secret to 20/20 Eyes

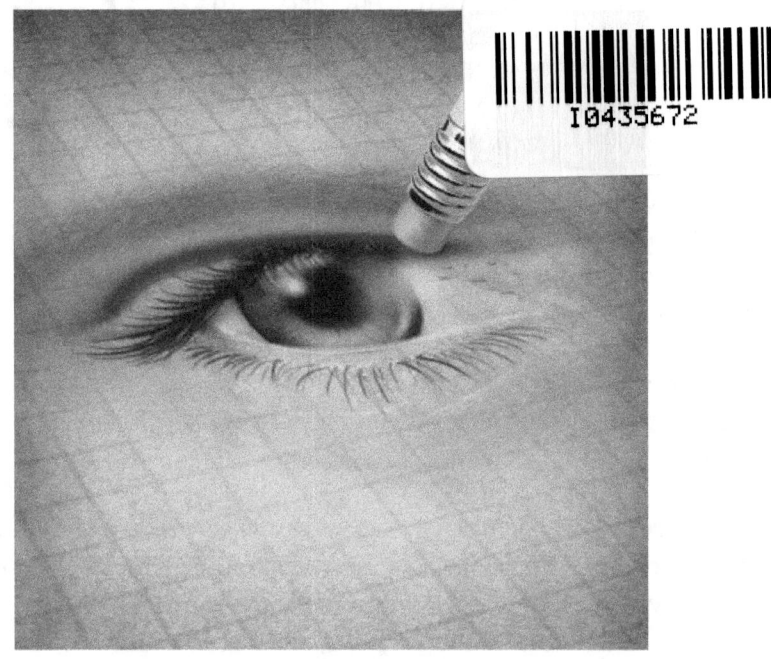

Health Learning Series

M. Usman

Mendon Cottage Books

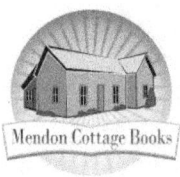

JD-Biz Publishing

Disclaimer

The information is this book is provided for informational purposes only. It is not intended to be used and medical advice or a substitute for proper medical treatment by a qualified health care provider. The information is believed to be accurate as presented based on research by the author.

The contents have not been evaluated by the U.S. Food and Drug Administration or any other Government or Health Organization and the contents in this book are not to be used to treat cure or prevent disease.

The author or publisher is not responsible for the use or safety of any diet, procedure or treatment mentioned in this book. The author or publisher is not responsible for errors or omissions that may exist.

Warning

The Book is for informational purposes only and before taking on any diet, treatment or medical procedure, it is recommended to consult with your primary health care provider.

Our books are available at

1. Amazon.com
2. Barnes and Noble
3. Itunes
4. Kobo
5. Smashwords
6. Google Play Books

Table of Contents

Vision 4
    Chapter # 1: An Introduction 4
    Chapter # 2: The Eye 6
    Chapter # 3: Eye Under-Stress 9
    Chapter # 4: Facts & Misconceptions 11
    Chapter # 5: Signs & Symptoms 16
A Healthy Diet 17
Recipes 24
    Chapter # 1: Turkey Burgers with Orange Peppers 24
    Chapter # 2: Pumpkin Mousse 26
    Chapter # 3: Roasted Salmon & Melon Salsa 27
    Chapter # 4: Chicken Almond Wraps 28
    Chapter # 5: Balsamic Chicken 30
    Chapter # 6: Chocolate Chip Pancakes 31
    Chapter # 7: Apricot Chicken 33
Conclusion 34
References 35
Author Bio 36
Publisher 47

Vision

Chapter # 1: An Introduction

Can you imagine a single day without your vision? I think every person on this world who has been blessed with vision would answer "No" to that.

Eyes are one of the most complex, fragile, and vital organs of our body that nature has bestowed on us. They are one of the most reliable sources to gather information from the surroundings and are one of the 5 senses that form a human body. But, with the passage of time the dexterity of our eyes start to decline and soon one's vision becomes sluggish. Interestingly, the decline of one's vision is not much related to age; a young adult for that matter could have a fast declining eye sight for a multitude of reasons. A visit to an optician can reveal that, and soon you'll be prescribed a pair of glasses to help correct your vision. The glasses would undoubtedly help correct your vision, but the bitter truth about them is that you'll get addicted to them and find it very hard to see without them. Research has clearly shown that vision aids only perform the job of "assisting" your eyes and not actually improving their vision in the long term.

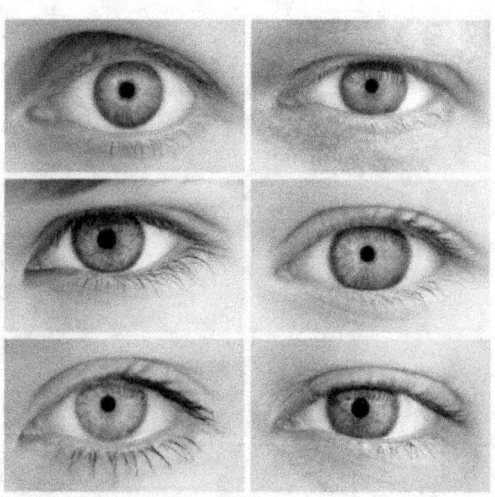

What is vision, exactly?

People use the word "vision" several times without even really knowing its meaning. It is commonly used in conjunction with "seeing" or "ability to see"; but that's not the whole definition.

A vision is your ability to perceive what's around you. It's not just the ability to see colors, shapes and objects, but a way to capture the living essence of the world around you. The humans are blessed with five senses and each work together to give you that perfect input. If your eyes were removed from the equation your vision would be hugely dented and the result would be something that would nowhere be close to the real thing.

Chapter # 2: The Eye

The Eye is the primary organ responsible for our "vision" and before we dive right into how the eye performs its functions, it would be best to state its anatomy. As you read the text, you'll be astonished by how the eye co-ordinates with the brain to provide such unique, accurate, and vivid pictures of the outside world. There are many parts of the eye that enable it to perform its function, and even though you don't need to have a sound knowledge of all of them, it sure wouldn't hurt you to know how they all work together to provide you with the gift of vision.

- **Cornea:**

  The Cornea is a translucent covering whose task is to transmit as well as focus the incoming light.

- **Fovea:**

  It is located right at the center of the macula and is responsible for providing you with sharp vision.

- **Iris:**

  It is that part of the eye that is tasked with the regulation of the amount of light that gets into the eye; it is also colored. In bright light, the iris is responsible for contracting the pupil so the amount of light getting in can be reduced while in low light conditions is expands so that more light could enter into the eye.

- **Lens:**

  The lens is transparent in appearance and is responsible for re-directing the light input to the back of the eye. The condition of the lens gets worse over time; cataracts are one of the biggest problems faced due to bad lens.

- **Macula:**

  Macula is another part of the eye that deteriorates with age. It is found in the retina and it contains light sensitive cells. These cells are the main reason behind how we view the tiniest of details so perfectly.

- **Optic nerve:**

  This nerve is made up of millions of nervous fibers that allow the transmission of messages from the retina to the brain. These signals are received by the brain which processes them to give us our vision.

- **Pupil:**

  It is the less-lighter opening located right in the center of the iris; the pupil contracts or dilates depending on the lighting conditions in the environment.

- **Retina:**

  It is the nerve that lines at the backside of the eye. The light that enters into the eye is directed into the retina which sends them to the brain in the form of electric impulses.

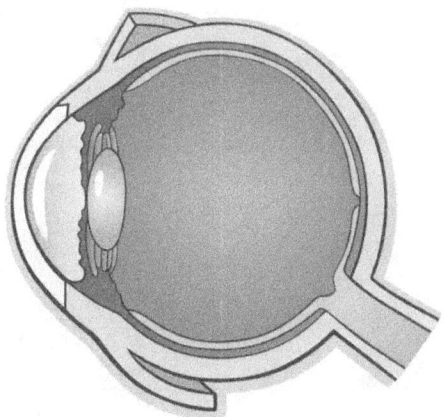

All parts of the eye work together to give you perfect vision; if any one of them lags behind, the final image is affected. Quite often, the human eye is compared to a digital camera and to some extent this analogy is not wrong:

1. The cornea is responsible for focusing on the incoming light, the same way a camera's lens does.

2.   When light enters the cornea, it is passed on to the iris which is similar to diaphragm in a camera.

3.   The lens of the eye automatically focuses on objects near or far, similar to the auto-focus feature in a camera.

4.   The electronic image sensor in a camera that carry outs the light captured by the lens onto the electronic parts works similar to the retina that conveys the light sensations onto the brain.

5.   The electric signals are then transmitted onto the brain; the visual cortex is ultimately responsible for our vision.

Another very interesting term used with respect to vision is the "field of view"; it is the extent to which the eye can capture its surroundings at a particular moment. The placement of the eyes in this regard determines how much the eye can see. Many birds have 360 degrees vision which means they can see their front, back and sides, but humans only have 180 degrees limited vision. Several eye diseases can actually restrict this vision and degrade it, limiting the person's ability to see.

Chapter # 3: Eye Under-Stress

Many muscles work in conjunction to give the eye a balanced and functioning vision. When these muscles come under stress, the first sensation that the body feels is stress. Strain in the eyes is an easy way to preemptively diagnose potential problems with one's vision and correct them before they start causing real issues.

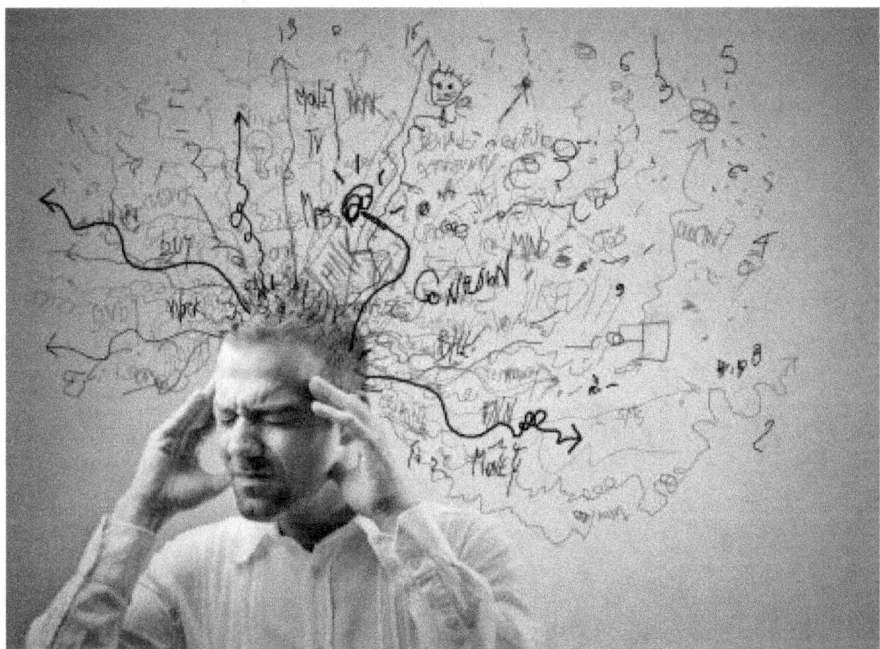

In a nutshell, eye strain is a discomfort that you feel in the eyes after you perform a gruesome task that involves focusing the eye in and out for a long period of time. There is no doubt about it that eye strain is uncomfortable in addition to being annoying, but it's harmless in most cases and diminishes after some rest is given. Nevertheless, there is always a possibility that eye strain might mean something other than just fatigue; it might mean that the eye is getting too tired and can't work the same way it used to.

Poor health is the biggest factor that plays a role of causing eye strain. This along with several other factors begins to cause problems in the eye that no longer remain limited to strain or annoyance. Often, lifestyle factors can be traced all the way back to childhood when a child faces the pressure of keeping up with his/her classmates. In addition, a child may have developed poor habits since then, which could be causing problems. More scientific evidence is revealing that as soon as a child starts going to school, his/her eyesight starts to worsen. More factors that can contribute to bad eye-sight are:

- Focusing for too long – If you focus on an object for a long period of time, soon you'll start experiencing eye strain. This is exactly why your eyes are made in a way so that they keep shifting focus from near to far instead of just being static at one focal length.

- Poor lighting – Poor lighting conditions forces the eyes to work harder than it normally does which increases strain on the eyes.

- Glare – Glare, direct or indirect can cause problems for the eyes. Direct glare is obtained from a light source that shines directly upon the eye while indirect glare is given off reflections from screens.

Chapter # 4: Facts & Misconceptions

A person's eye sight is affected by a number of factors including poor lifestyle, diet, etc. In this society, many people tend to have their own theories as to what causes poor vision. Some of them right, most of them wrong! While the wrong one's have no affect over our vision, they do play tricks on our mind; we worry about them more and try to fix these problem, but unfortunately no real benefit is seen as all these "advices" and "theories" are just hoaxes. It is thus very necessary that these myths be busted and person be guided correctly about his/her vision.

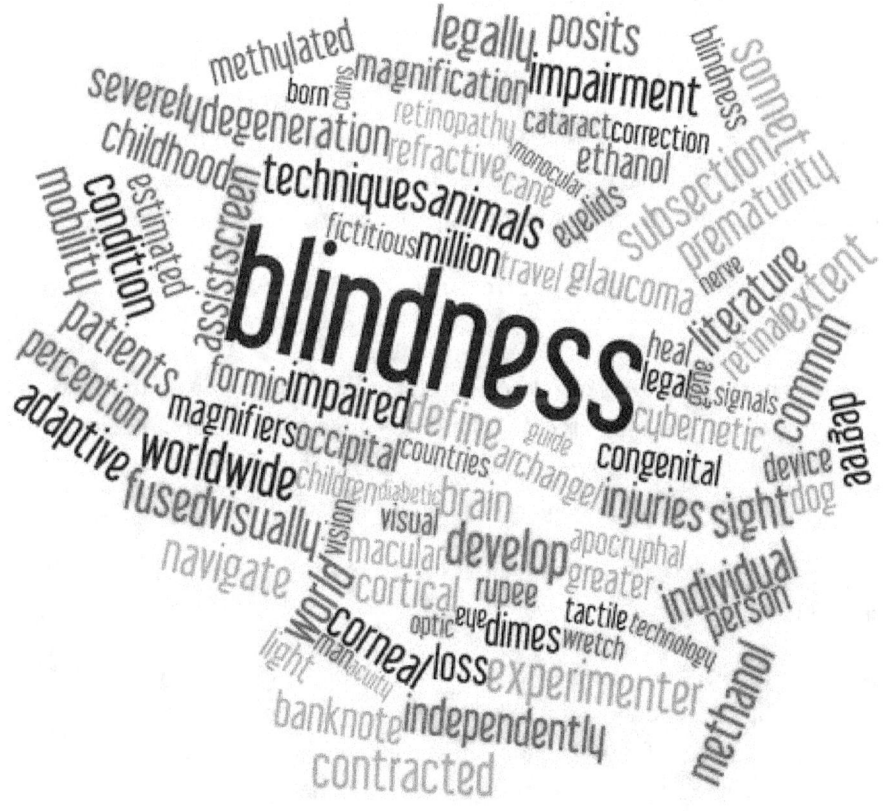

Firstly, the myths about eye-sight and vision are discussed followed by the facts.

Myth # 1 – Glasses will improve your eyesight:

This is not true. Research has actually shown that eyesight can actually get worse with the use of glasses. Eyes have the natural tendency to heal themselves if they are given proper care as well as attention. A combination of proper nutritional intake, eye exercises, as well as common sense, can go a long way.

Myth # 2 – Dim light is harmful for the eyes:

This needs to be put to rest right away! Reading in dim light puts stress to your eyes, but does not immediately causes damage to the eyes. This stress, along with the other factors, overtime causes damage.

Myth # 3 – Carrots Heal Vision!

Carrots are undoubtedly a rich source of vitamin A which is required for healthy vision, but this does not mean that consumption of huge quantities of carrots can lead to a mass improvement in one's vision. A good amount of vitamin A can also be absorbed from other parts of diet as well!

Myth # 4 – Your eyes will get worse over time and there's nothing you can do about it!

This is plain wrong. Our eyes are amazing organs and just like other parts of the body, they need to be treated with care. Unfortunately, their health is taken for-granted which results in loss of vision. But, if a person carries out a healthy regimen, he/she can have perfect vision up until death.

Myth # 5 – Eye examinations must be taken only when an irregularity is noticed.

An eye examination reveals the current health of the eye. If any part of the eye is losing its functions, it can be spotted way before it permanently becomes disabled. If a person takes tests only when he/she notices something wrong, the eye exam won't fix it and he would have to undergo treatment anyway.

Myth # 6 – Computer screens are harmful for the eye.

No, computer screens do not cause damage to the eyes. Ultraviolet rays and x-rays cause problems for the eyes, but these are not emitted by computer screens; not even CRT monitors. They put unneeded strain on the eyes but that's the extent of it.

Myth # 7 – Watching the TV too closely damages the eyes.

A child is much better at seeing things closer to the eyes, i.e. focusing closely rather than seeing farther objects. This is why children usually read books close to their eyes. This habit diminishes with time but if it doesn't, the child must undergo an eye exam.

Myth # 8 – People with a weaker vision should avoid looking at things with great detail.

It is a well-known misconception that looking at things that contain great detail can inflict further damage to one's eyes. This concept is based on an analogy that the eye is a muscle which will become weak if put under constant strain. A better analogy is that of a camera; cameras don't wear out if they constantly take pictures with great detail.

Myth # 9 – Eyes can be transplanted.

At the current stage of scientific development, this is not possible. The eyes are connected to our brain with an optic nerve, which once severed, can never recover. Therefore what happens during an eye replacement surgery is that the cornea undergoes transplantations and not the eye. This is often misunderstood.

Myth # 10 – Contact lenses improve one's eyesight.

Contact lenses are just like glasses; instead they fit right into the eye. They provide temporary relief but in no way are the final answer. Wearing contact lenses for a long time can actually cause more damage like:

i.   They may cause the eyes to dry excessively.

ii. They may cause corneal infections.

iii. They may cause scratches in the eye.

iv. They can cause inflammation.

v.   They may force the shape of the cornea to change.

vi.   They may start an allergic reaction.

At this stage you would be quite familiar with what's right and what's not. The facts with respect to eye sight are as follows:

- ✓ Problems related to vision are the second most common health problems found in the US; they affect over 120 million people across the country.

- ✓ Around 61 percent of the American population makes use of some medical correction technique to achieve greater vision. In numbers, 61% makes up almost 172 million people. Moreover, a majority of these people are not even aware that they can have better vision with a healthy diet.

- ✓ People who repeatedly visit their optician for not being able to see clearly are unaware of the fact that glasses don't help their vision; they actually play a negative role.

- ✓ One out of 4 children in the US between the ages of 3 and 16 wear glasses for better vision.

- ✓ Around 75 percent of the people who rely on their computers most of the days develop some kind of vision problem; symptoms range from dry eyes, blurred vision to headaches.

- ✓ Cataracts are one of the most self-reported vision problems and are the third leading cause of blindness.

If you remember the time you were prescribed with glasses, you would also remember being instructed by your parents to keep wearing them so your eyes can adjust to them. And once you get adjusted to them, everything else looks blurry and you experience headaches if you don't wear the glasses anymore. There is only one possible explanation to this, i.e. your eyesight is actually deteriorating over time.

The human body is designed to heal itself and over time with proper nutrition, it does. The addition of manual methods like glasses and lenses ultimately damage the natural sanctity of our body. There is no doubt that science has helped mankind in a lot of ways and has accelerated repair mechanisms; still it does not provide the body with a perfect replacement.

Over 90 percent of the information received by our brain comes from the eyes. It is unarguably the most important receptive channel. If it weren't for the eye our ability to judge would be affected and with that, everything else too; thus it is vital that we take care of our eyes in the best possible manner.

Chapter # 5: Signs & Symptoms

Now that every fact and myth has been cleared up and you know all about how the eye works, it's time to tell you about the signs that appear when your eye sight starts to decline. The following are the signs that a person with deteriorating vision would experience:

1. Blurred vision,

2. Burning or itching in the eyes,

3. Double vision,

4. Sore eyes,

5. Shoulder pain,

6. Neck pain,

7. Frequent headaches,

8. Heightened sensitivity to light,

The effect of eye strain may appear to vanish as you let your eyes rest, but repeated episodes of eye stress means something else; your vision is no longer perfect.

A Healthy Diet

Nutrition plays a central role in governing the health of your vision. It has been at the center of research for quite some time now and studies have shown that particular foods have very positive effects on the vision. Scientists are also interested in finding out how vitamins and minerals influence eyes and prevent against diseases like cataracts and AMD. A good, well-balanced diet is not just vital for the eye but for the whole human body.

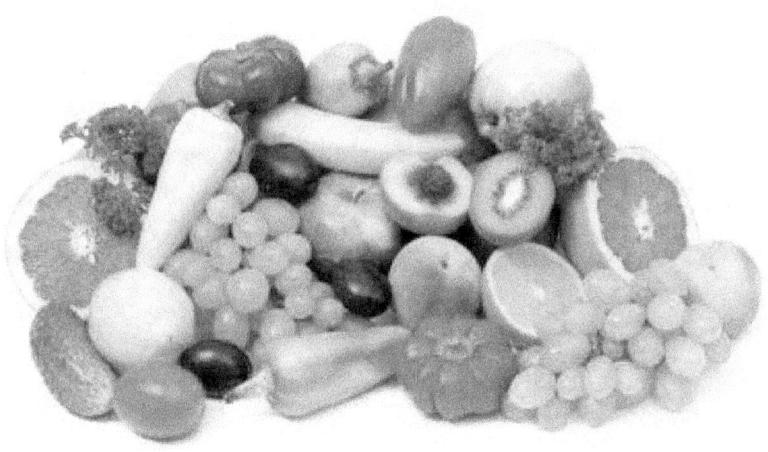

One of the most notable examples of a healthy diet warding off ailments is that of *xeraphthalamia*, a condition common in individuals in developing countries. It is known to strike during childhood and cause blindness. This condition is caused due to lack of Vitamin A in the body which can be fulfilled eating fresh vegetables and meat. But, as developing countries don't have the required mechanism to provide adequate nutrition to the whole populace, the disease strikes.

Studies have revealed that antioxidants can greatly boost vision and protect them from harmful compounds. The most important vitamins known for their antioxidant ability are vitamins A, C and E. They are found in many vegetables and fruits and should be in a person's regular intake.

- Brussels' Sprouts,

- Grapefruit,

- Dried Apricots,

- Green Leafy Vegetables,

- Green Beans,

- Kiwis,

- Green Peas,

- Carrots,

- Tomatoes,

- Peppers,

- Oranges,

These antioxidants are also found in dairy products like eggs, milk, butter, seeds, and nuts.

Furthermore, there are two particular types of antioxidants known as carotenoids that have repeatedly shown the ability to decrease the risk of age-related macular degeneration. The antioxidants called Zeaxanthin and lutein are found in fruits and vegetables like:

- Mangoes,

- Green vegetables,

- Bilberries,

- Yellow peppers,

- Spinach,

- Tangerines,

- Broccoli,

- Oranges,

- Lettuce,

- Eggs,

- Corn

Seeing each vitamin individually, vitamin A is probably the most important one. It is very vital for attaining clear vision and is responsible for protecting the cornea. Vitamin A drops are commonly used to treat dry eyes. It has also shown effectiveness against inflammatory conditions, and is known to reduce the risk of macular degeneration.

Foods rich in vitamin A include:

- Carrots,

- Sweet potatoes,

- Leafy vegetables,

- Romaine lettuce

- Dried apricots

- Squash

- Cantaloupe melons

- Red peppers

- Mangoes

- Tuna fish

Another very effective vitamin is Vitamin C which keeps the eye healthy by protecting it against UV light damage. Vitamin C helps prevent the development of cataracts, which causes the lens of an eye to get blurry and respond unusually to light. Most people in the US follow a minimum requirement for vitamin C which ranges from 75 mg for women to 90 mg for men.

Foods rich in Vitamin C include:

- Brussels sprouts,

- Broccoli,

- Kohlrabi,

- Guava,

- Pineapple,

- Papaya,

- Red bell peppers,

- Raspberries,

- Strawberries

Vitamin E is a fat soluble vitamin which helps in preventing both macular degeneration as well as cataracts. Vitamin E is found in abundance in the following foods:

- Cottonseed oil,

- Almonds,

- Papaya,

- Hazelnuts,

- Peanut butter,

- Sunflower oil,

- Wheat germ,

- Wheat germ oil,

- Sunflower seeds Kernels,

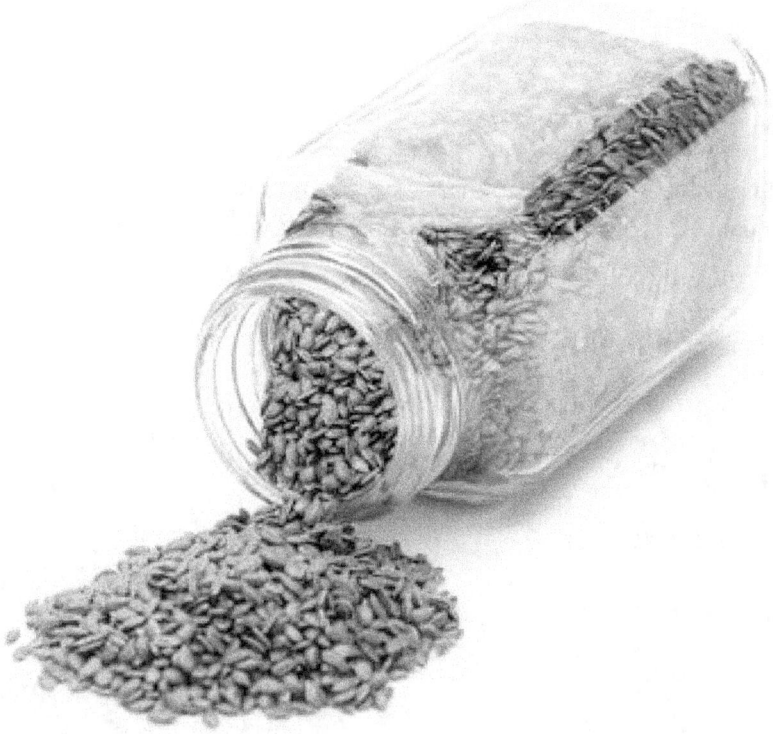

A mineral which plays a huge role in the maintenance of the eyes is zinc. It is found in great concentrations in the eye and is vital for a healthy retina. The requirement for this mineral increase as a person ages and it is thus important for a person to consume zinc regularly. Foods rich in zinc include:

- Black eyed peas,

- Almonds,

- Chicken,

- Brown rice,

- Milk,

- Ground beef,

- Garbanzo beans,

- Tofu,

- Wheat germ,

- Sunflower seeds,

Beta carotene is a compound that helps in night vision and keeps it at optimum levels. Beta carotene supplements are widely available in markets but there are many foods rich in it too:

- Beet greens,

- Carrots,

- Cantaloupe Melons,

- Apricots,

- Kale,

- Collard greens,

- Red bell peppers,

- Romaine lettuce,

- Spinach,

- Turnip greens,

- Winter squash,

- Sweet potatoes,

- Papaya

Recipes

Chapter # 1: Turkey Burgers with Orange Peppers

Makes 4 servings

Ingredients:

- 1 pound extra-lean ground turkey

- 1 egg

- ½ cup chopped green onions

- ¼ cup whole wheat bread crumbs

- ¼ cup flat-leaf parsley, chopped

- Salt & pepper

For the toppings:

- 4 whole wheat buns (burger)

- 2 orange peppers

- 3 tablespoon Dijon mustard

- Leaf lettuce

For the onions:

- 2 yellow onions

- Olive oil

Directions:

Firstly, mix all the ingredients required for the burgers and shape them into patties. Place each of the prepared patties on a sheet of parchment paper and place it in a refrigerator. Next, preheat the grill to high heat; place the peppers on it and keep it turning until all sides are charred. Remove the peppers from the grill and place them in a pepper bag. Close it tightly and let it cool for about 10 – 15 minutes. The steam that accumulates in the bag will help the skin separate from the peppers making them easier to peel. Once the peppers are cool enough, peel them, remove the stems, and white membranes. Mix 1 tablespoon of the pepper juice with 3 tablespoons of Dijon mustard and set aside the roasted wedges. Flip the turkey patties onto the grill and cook each side until desired wellness achieved. When the patties are almost ready, toast the burger buns on the grill. To finally assemble, spread the mustard-mixture on the buns, followed by the pepper wedges and the patty. Top it all up with a leaf lettuce.

If you can, prepare caramelized onions by cooking thinly sliced onions over medium heat and olive oil for 20 minutes; seasoning them with salt.

Chapter # 2: Pumpkin Mousse

Makes 4 servings

Ingredients:

- 1 envelope gelatin

- 1 cup pumpkin puree (240 grams)

- ½ cup maple syrup

- ½ teaspoon mixed spice

- ¼ cup orange juice

- ½ cup Greek yogurt

- ¼ cup whipping cream

- ½ teaspoon mixed spices (cinnamon, nutmeg, ginger, clove, etc.)

Directions:

In a large bowl, mix the yogurt and pumpkin using a whisk. Sprinkle the gelatin with the juice and set it aside for 3 minutes so that the maple syrup could get ready. Bring the maple-syrup to a boil on medium heat and while stirring constantly, let it heat. Pour this boiling syrup over the orange juice until the gelatin melts and mix it well using a whisk. Add spices and orange zest into the mixture and combine. In a chilled bowl, whip the cream so that firm peaks begin to form. Use a mixer to whip the mixes for about a minute and finally fold the cream onto the pumpkin mixture with the help of a spatula. Ladle this mixture into serving cups and chill in a freezer for about 3 hours.

Chapter # 3: Roasted Salmon & Melon Salsa

Makes 4 servings

Ingredients:

- 4 wild, frozen and fresh salmon fillets

- 1 tablespoon olive oil

- Salt and pepper

- 1 cup cantaloupe in ¼ in. cubes

- ½ red pepper in ¼ in. cubes

- 1 green onion

- 1 tablespoon cilantro, fresh

- Juice and Zest

- 1 tablespoon olive oil

Directions:

Preheat a broiler to maximum or 400 degrees. Use aluminum foil to line a cooking sheet. Place the fish fillets on the sheet and brush them up with olive oil. Sprinkle a little pepper and some salt on each fillet and place them in the oven for 5-10 minutes or until they are brown and cooked properly.

While the salmon is still cooking, mix the green onion, cilantro, cantaloupe, and red pepper and season it with salt and pepper. In a bowl, whisk the lime zest, juice, and olive oil. Pour this dressing over the salsa and mix them to combine. When the salmon is done, place a fillet on a plate, and add in ¼ spoon of salsa on the top, serving with brown rice and green salad.

Chapter # 4: Chicken Almond Wraps

Makes 4 servings

Ingredients:

- 1 tablespoon olive oil or canola oil

- 1 cup frozen peas

- 2 skinless, boneless chicken breasts (cook them and shred in to pieces)

- 1 chopped orange pepper

- 1 large orange (peeled, quartered and sliced)

- 2 green onions

- ¼ cup fresh cilantro, chopped

- ¼ cup sliced almonds

- Leaf lettuce

- Romaine lettuce

For the sauce:

- 2 teaspoons rice vinegar

- 4 tablespoons almond butter

- 4 teaspoons soy sauce

- 3 teaspoons honey

- Hot water

- Dash hot sauce

Directions:

Mix the peas, pepper, poultry, orange, green onion, cilantro and almonds in a bowl and set aside. In a separate bowl, combine the rice vinegar, almond butter, honey, soy sauce, and hot sauce. Add 2 tablespoons of water and keep stirring it. If the sauce is too thick, add in one more tablespoon of water and continue to do so until the sauce is consistently thick. Use two tablespoons of this sauce to dress the poultry mix and toss it gently to combine. Separate the leftover dipping sauce into a bowl for each individual. Spoon the prepared chicken mixture onto kale leaf or lettuce and fold it. Finally, serve with dipping sauce.

Chapter # 5: Balsamic Chicken

Makes 4 servings

Ingredients:

- 2 large sliced red bell peppers

- 1 large yellow onion

- ¼ teaspoons red pepper

- 4 cloves minced garlic

- 4 six-ounce skinless, boneless pieces of chicken breast

- ¼ teaspoon Kosher salt

- 1/3 cup balsamic vinegar

- ¼ teaspoons black pepper

- 1x 15 ounce can of diced tomatoes

Directions:

Coat a medium – large sized sauté pan with oil spray and heat it over high heat. Add the bell peppers and onions and sauté for 5 more minutes or until the vegetables start to soften. Add a tablespoon of water and additional oil spray if you feel that the vegetables are starting to stick to the bottom. Add garlic powder or garlic along with red pepper flakes and sauté for 1 more minute, while stirring it constantly. Season the breasts with salt and pepper as desired and add them to a pan, cooking for 4 minutes on both sides. Add the canned tomatoes and balsamic vinegar and reduce the heat to medium, simmering for 25 minutes. Finally season with salt and serve.

Chapter # 6: Chocolate Chip Pancakes

Makes 6 servings

Ingredients:

- ½ cup whole-wheat flour

- ¼ cup unsweetened cocoa

- ½ cup all-purpose flour

- ¼ cup sugar

- 1 ½ teaspoons baking powder

- 2 tablespoons ground flax

- 1 teaspoon salt

- 1 large egg

- 1 egg white

- 1 cup fat free milk

- 1 tablespoon canola oil

- ½ cup semisweet chocolate chips

- 1 dollop nonfat yogurt

- 1 squirt whipped topping

- 1 sprinkling chocolate shaving

Directions:

In a well sized mixing bowl, whisk the cocoa, sugar, flours, baking powder, flaxseeds, and salt. In a medium sized bowl, beat the eggs and add oil, milk, and vanilla, whisking until combined. Pour the wet ingredients into the dry ones and stir until the newly formed batter is blended and not even a single dry streak remains. Delicately add in the chocolate chips and be sure not to mix it too much as this will cause the pancakes to become chewy. If time allows you, rest the batter for 10 more minutes before starting to cook the pancakes.

Cook the pancakes for about 1 to 2 minutes, or until small bubbles appear at the edges. Flip the pancakes and cook for one more minute or until the center is adequately cooked. Coat the skillet yet again with oil spray between batches in order to prevent the pancakes from sticking. Add your desired toppings and enjoy!

Chapter # 7: Apricot Chicken

Makes 4 servings

Ingredients:

- 4 small apricots, diced into ½ in. chunks

- 4x 4 ounce skinless chicken breasts

- Kosher salt

- Black pepper

- 1 teaspoon light brown sugar

- 1 teaspoon agave nectar

- ½ cup unsweetened applesauce

Directions:

Preheat a grill. Mix the chicken with olive oil, season it, and set it aside. Take a sheet of foil paper and place the apricots in it. Sprinkle the apricots with light brown sugar, agave nectar, and applesauce. Fold the foil so that a pouch forms and place this foil on the preheated grill. Place the chicken cutlets on the grill and cook each side for 5 – 8 minutes or until there are grill marks on the chicken which indicate that the chicken breast is cooked all the way. After the chicken reaches 165 degrees Fahrenheit, remove them from the grill. Divide the toppings evenly among the freshly grilled chicken pieces and serve.

Conclusion

If you are currently lucky enough that you have 20/20 vision, don't let the thought that it will last forever cross your mind. Just like every other part of your body, your eyes need to be treated with care too. Therefore, to keep up with the pace of this life and have a perfect vision, make regular visits to your optician for eye exams and early detection of symptoms of eye problems. This will greatly increase the chances of you dodging an eye disease rather than treating it. Furthermore, don't ignore any sign of eye strain no matter how minor it is as it just might be an indication from your body that something is not right. If the sign persists visit your optician and straighten it out. Along with keeping yourself up to date, consume a well-balanced, nutritious diet that will provide the body with all the right vitamins and minerals to repair it.

Best of luck!

References

http://www.123rf.com/photo_14837727_vision-loss-ad-losing-eyesight-medical-health-care-concept-with-a-human-sight-organ-being-erased-by-.html?term=macular%20degeneration

http://nl.123rf.com/photo_14697991_set-van-6-real-verschillende-open-ogen--enorme-size--macro.html

http://nl.123rf.com/photo_14601371_medische-vector-illustratie-van-het-menselijk-oog-ball-cross-section.html?term=parts%20of%20eye

http://nl.123rf.com/photo_17765960_jonge-man-heeft-verwarring-in-zijn-hoofd.html?term=stress

http://nl.123rf.com/photo_16501008_abstract-woordwolk-voor-blindness-met-gerelateerde-tags-en-voorwaarden.html?term=cornea

http://www.fotolia.com/id/50892535

http://www.fotolia.com/id/58392273

Author Bio

Muhammad Usman is a distinguished medical graduate of Allama Iqbal medical college (AIMC). He is a professional writer who has been in the field for more than 4 years. During this time he has produced 10,000+ articles, blogs, and eBooks on various niches related to diseases, health, fitness, nutrition, and well-being. He is a regular contributor to several journals related to medicine and surgery. He is the editor of several journals and newspapers.

Check out some of the other JD-Biz Publishing books

Gardening Series on Amazon

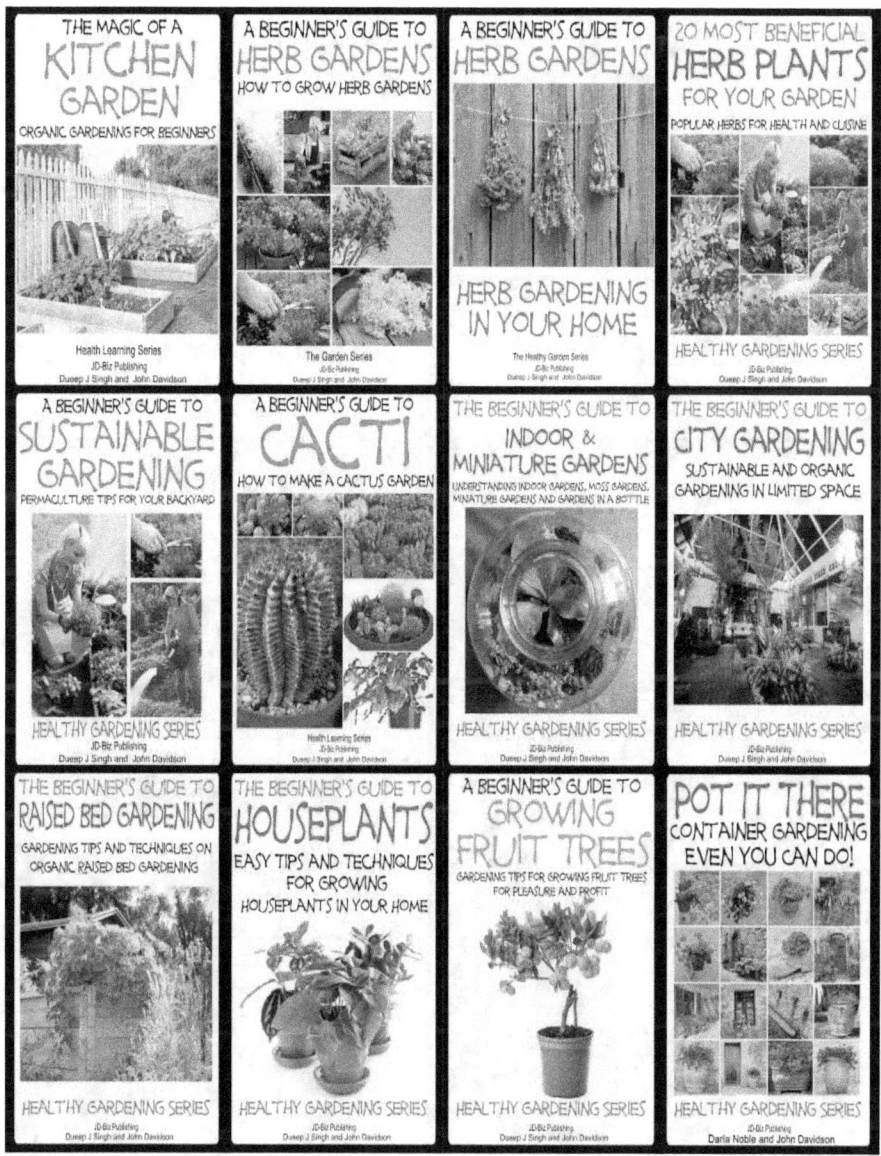

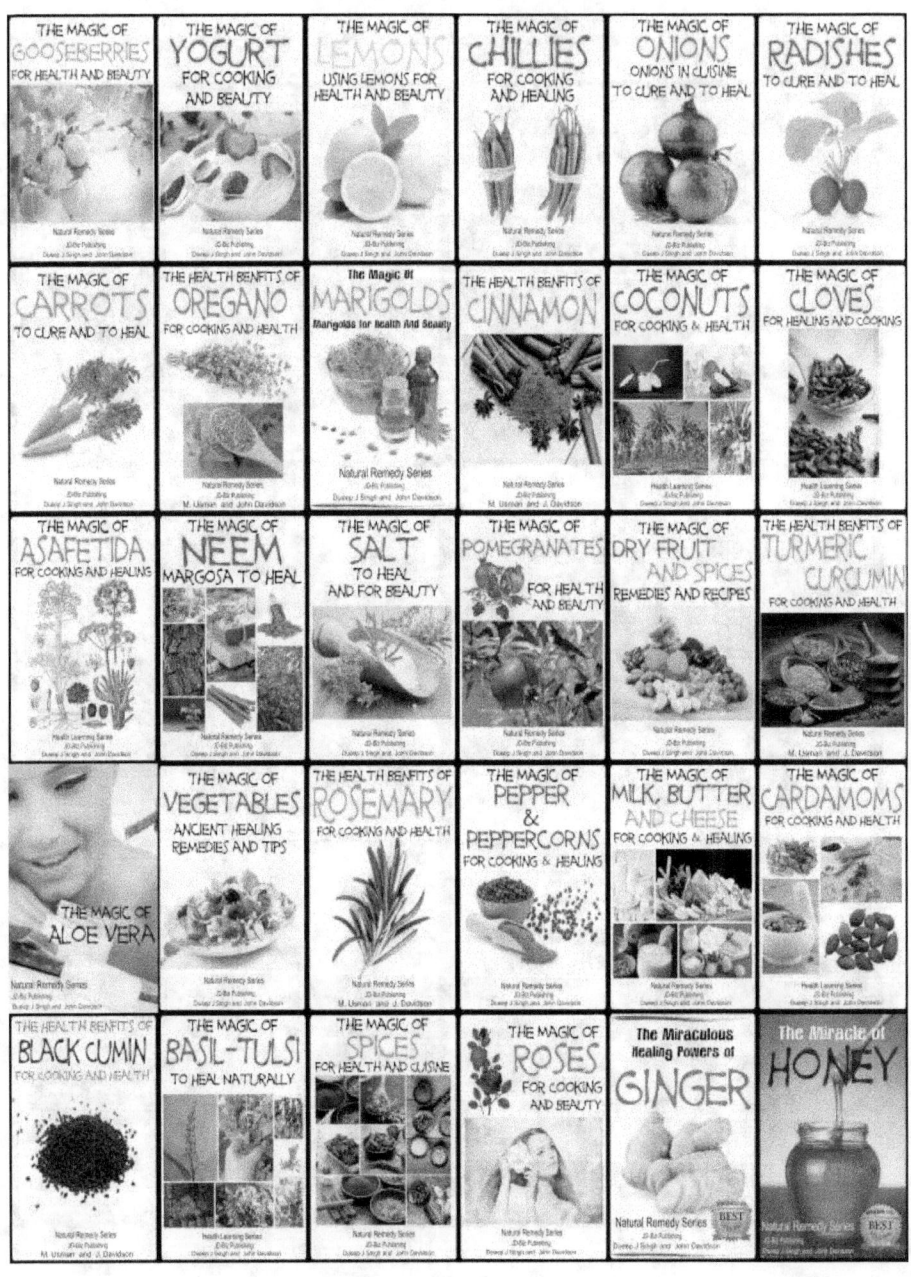

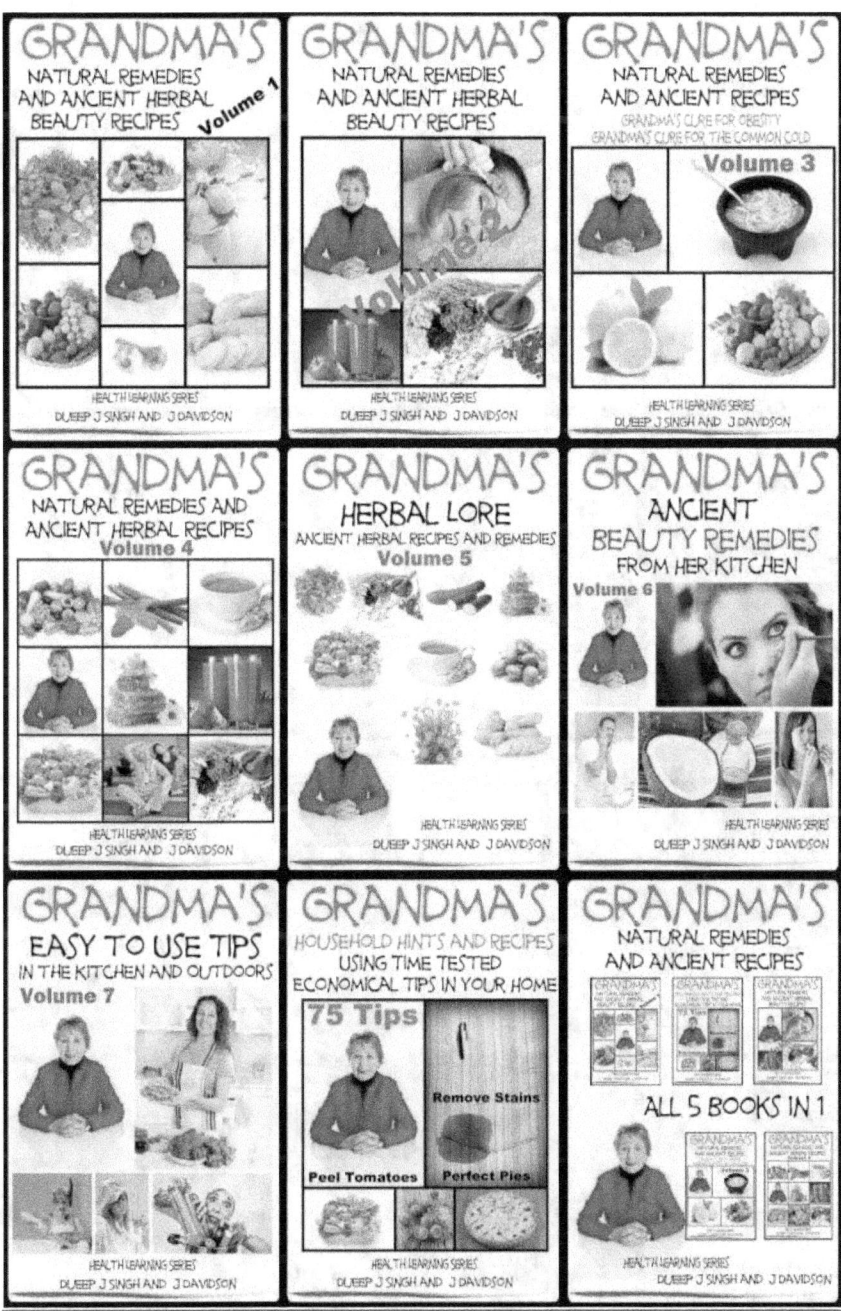

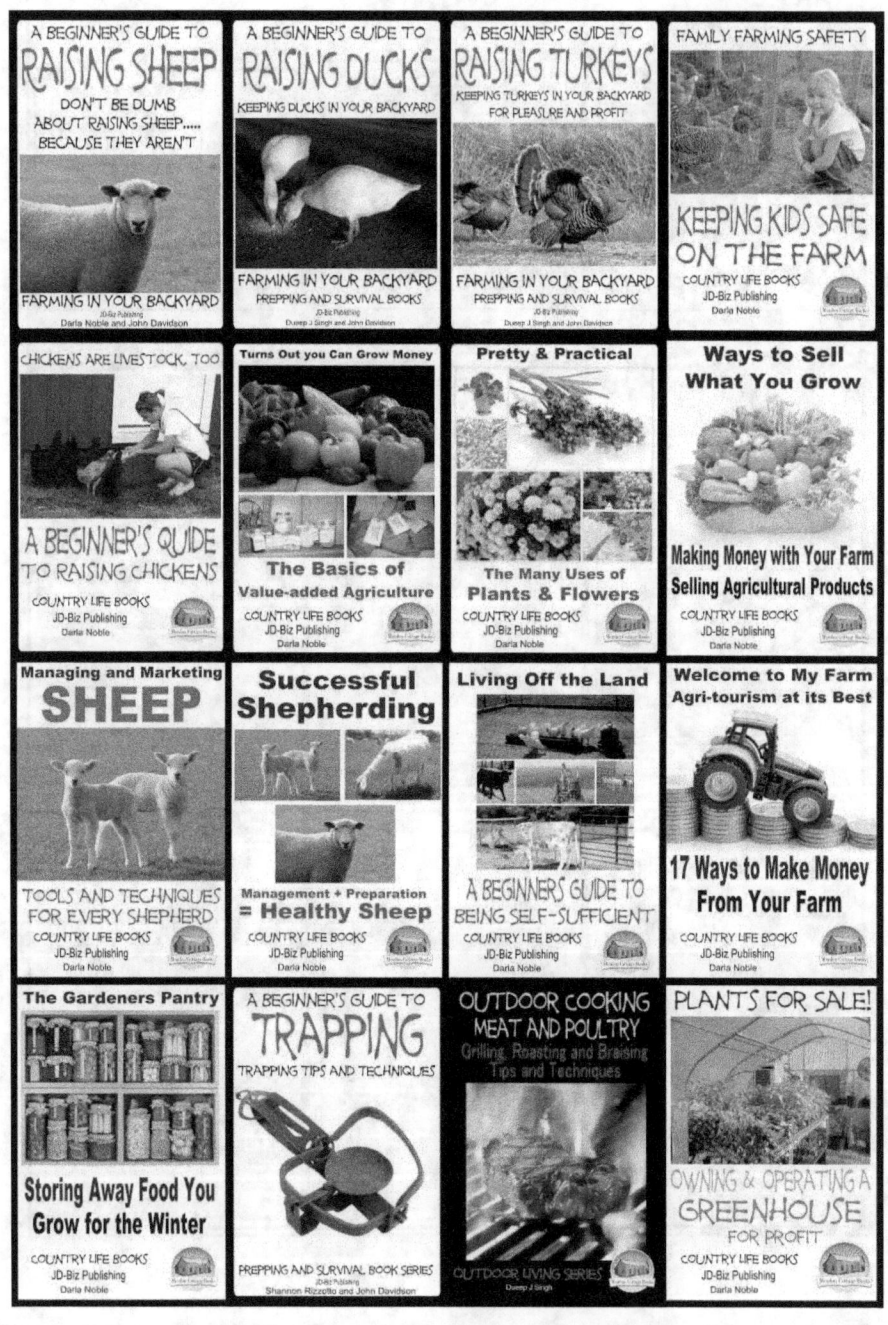

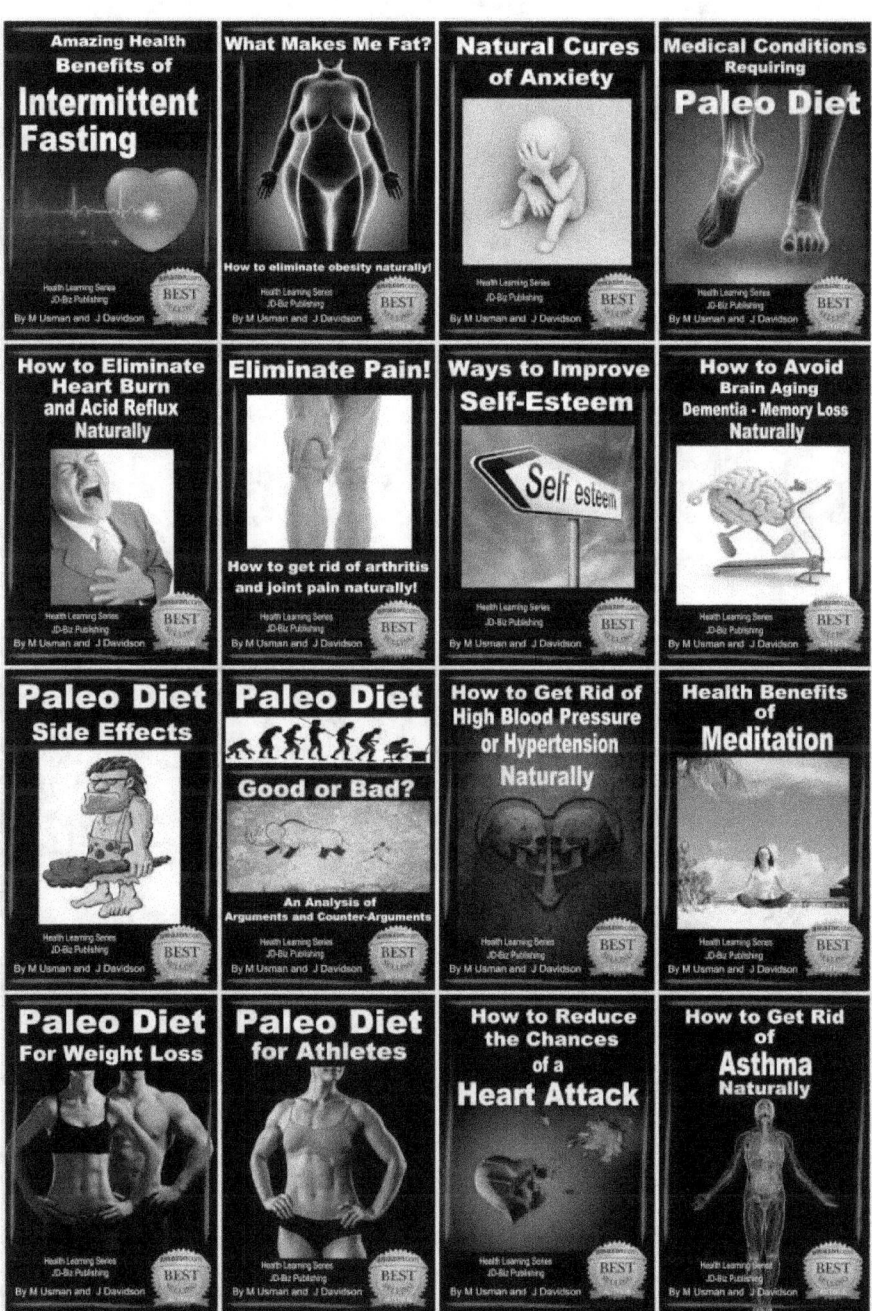

Amazing Animal Book Series

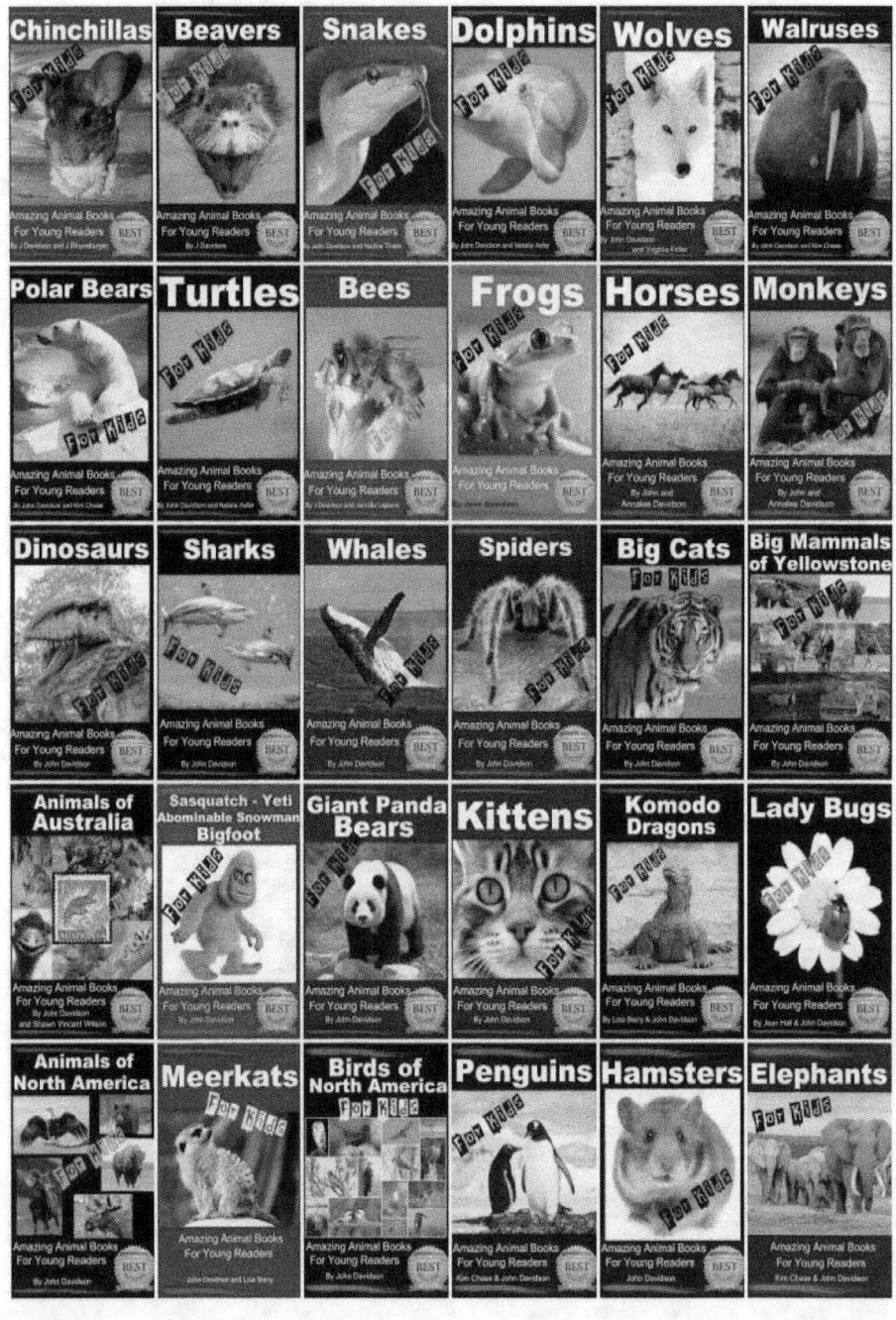

Learn To Draw Series

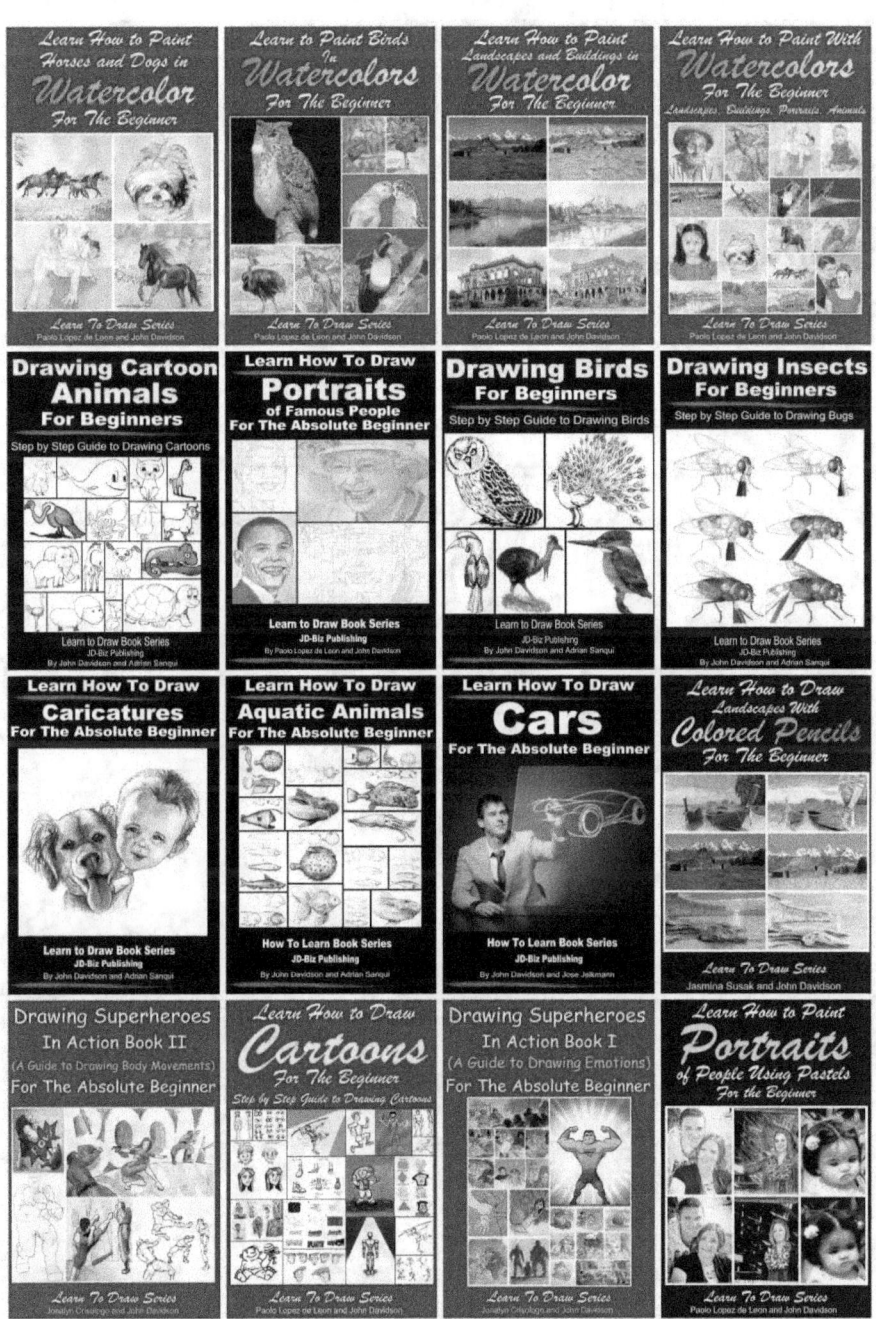

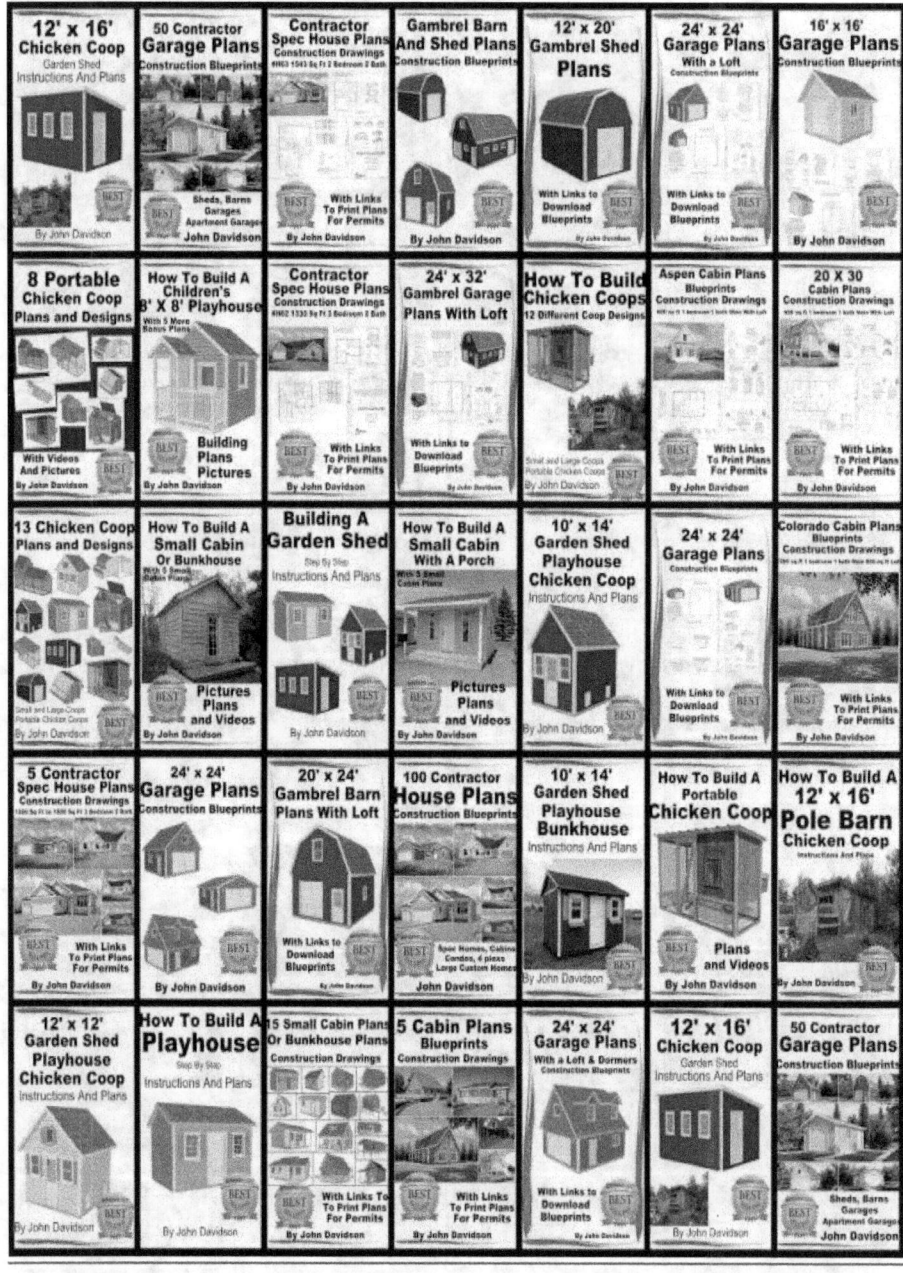

Entrepreneur Book Series

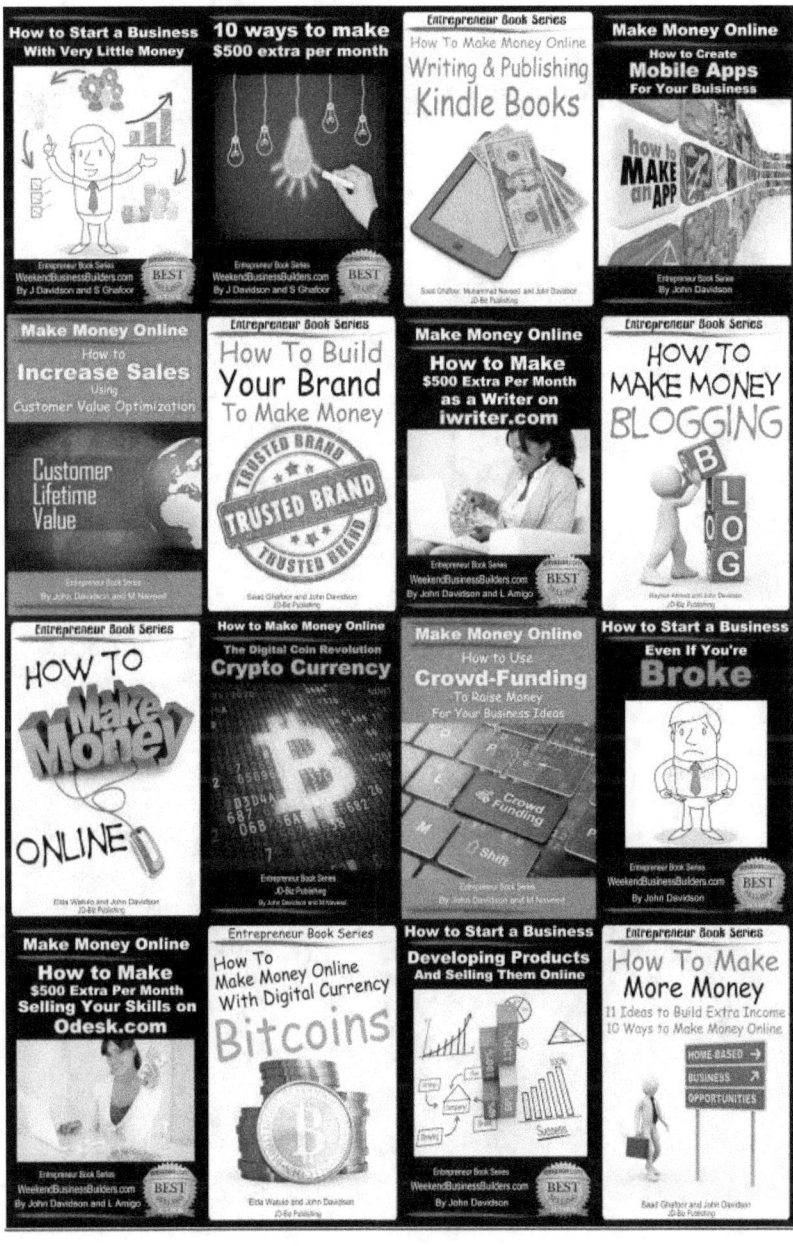

Our books are available at

1. Amazon.com

2. Barnes and Noble

3. Itunes

4. Kobo

5. Smashwords

6. Google Play Books

Publisher

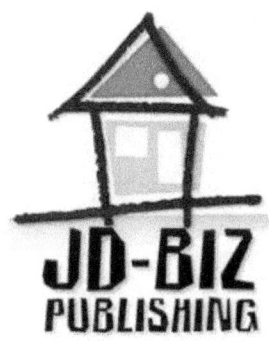

JD-Biz Corp

P O Box 374

Mendon, Utah 84325

http://www.jd-biz.com/

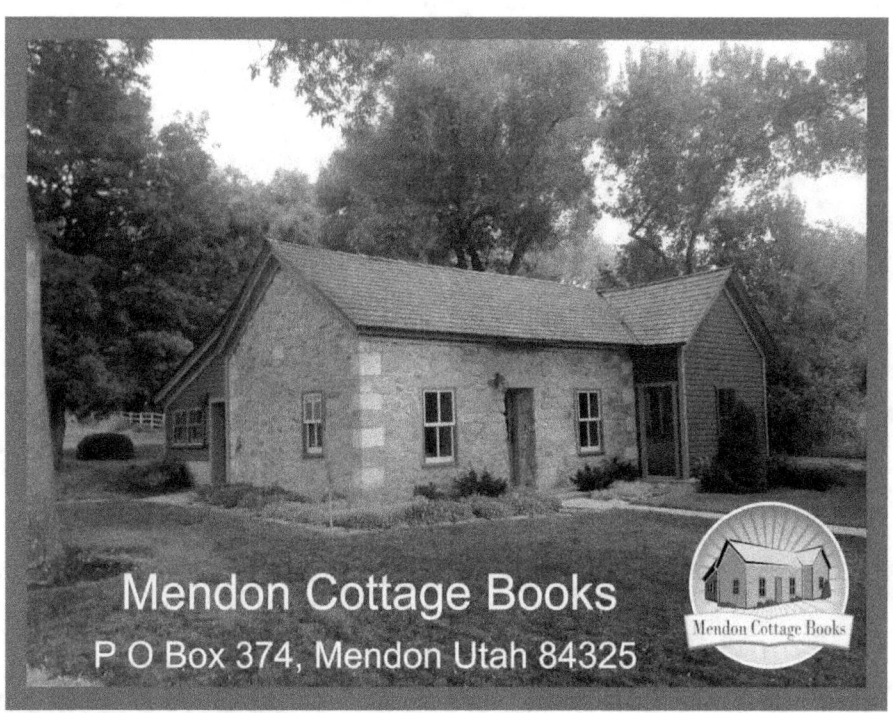

Mendon Cottage Books

P O Box 374, Mendon Utah 84325

www.ingramcontent.com/pod-product-compliance
Lightning Source LLC
Chambersburg PA
CBHW071142280526
45787CB00003B/1374